Contents

INTRODUCTION

In vitro fertilization (IVF) is a complex series of procedures used to help with fertility or prevent genetic problems and assist with the conception of a child.

During IVF, mature eggs are collected (retrieved) from ovaries and fertilized by sperm in a lab. Then the fertilized egg (embryo) or eggs (embryos) are transferred to a uterus. One full cycle of IVF takes about three weeks. Sometimes these steps are split into different parts and the process can take longer.

IVF is the most effective form of assisted reproductive technology. The procedure can be done using your own eggs and your partner's sperm. Or IVF may involve eggs, sperm or embryos from a known or anonymous donor. In some cases, a gestational carrier a woman who has an embryo implanted in her uterus might be used.

Your chances of having a healthy baby using IVF depend on many factors, such as your age and the cause of infertility. In addition, IVF can be time-consuming, expensive and invasive. If more than one embryo is transferred to your uterus, IVF can result in a pregnancy with more than one fetus (multiple pregnancy).

Your doctor can help you understand how IVF works, the potential risks and whether this method of treating infertility is right for you.

Why it's done

In vitro fertilization (IVF) is a treatment for infertility or genetic problems. If IVF is performed to treat infertility, you and your partner might be able to try less-invasive treatment options before attempting IVF, including fertility drugs to increase production of eggs or intrauterine insemination a procedure in which sperm are placed directly in your uterus near the time of ovulation.

Sometimes, IVF is offered as a primary treatment for infertility in women over age 40. IVF can also be done if you have certain health conditions. For example, IVF may be an option if you or your partner has:

Fallopian tube damage or blockage. Fallopian tube damage or blockage makes it difficult for an egg to be fertilized or for an embryo to travel to the uterus.

- Ovulation disorders.

If ovulation is infrequent or absent, fewer eggs are available for fertilization.

- Endometriosis.

Endometriosis occurs when the uterine tissue implants and grows outside of the uterus often affecting the function of the ovaries, uterus and fallopian tubes.

- Uterine fibroids.

Fibroids are benign tumors in the wall of the uterus and are common in women in their 30s and 40s. Fibroids can interfere with implantation of the fertilized egg.

- Previous tubal sterilization or removal.

If you've had tubal ligation a type of sterilization in which your fallopian tubes are cut or blocked to permanently prevent pregnancy and want to conceive, IVF may be an alternative to tubal ligation reversal.

- Impaired sperm production or function.

Below-average sperm concentration, weak movement of sperm (poor mobility), or abnormalities in sperm size and shape can make it difficult for sperm to fertilize an egg. If semen abnormalities are found, your partner might need to see a specialist to determine if there are correctable problems or underlying health concerns.

- Unexplained infertility.

Unexplained infertility means no cause of infertility has been found despite evaluation for common causes.

- A genetic disorder.

If you or your partner is at risk of passing on a genetic disorder to your child, you may be candidates for preimplantation genetic testing a procedure that involves IVF. After the eggs are harvested and fertilized, they're screened for certain genetic problems, although not all genetic problems can be found. Embryos that don't contain identified problems can be transferred to the uterus.

- Fertility preservation for cancer or other health conditions.

If you're about to start cancer treatment such as radiation or chemotherapy that could harm your fertility, IVF for fertility preservation may be an option. Women can have eggs harvested from their ovaries and frozen in an unfertilized state for later use. Or the eggs can be fertilized and frozen as embryos for future use.

Women who don't have a functional uterus or for whom pregnancy poses a serious health risk might choose IVF using another person to carry the pregnancy (gestational carrier). In this case, the woman's eggs are fertilized with sperm, but the resulting embryos are placed in the gestational carrier's uterus.

Risks

Risks of IVF include:

- Multiple births.

IVF increases the risk of multiple births if more than one embryo is transferred to your uterus. A pregnancy with multiple fetuses carries a higher risk of early labor and low birth weight than pregnancy with a single fetus does.

- Premature delivery and low birth weight.

Research suggests that IVF slightly increases the risk that the baby will be born early or with a low birth weight.

- Ovarian hyperstimulation syndrome.

Use of injectable fertility drugs, such as human chorionic gonadotropin (HCG), to induce ovulation can cause ovarian hyperstimulation syndrome, in which your ovaries become swollen and painful.

Symptoms typically last a week and include mild abdominal pain, bloating, nausea, vomiting and diarrhea. If you become pregnant, however, your symptoms might last several weeks. Rarely, it's possible to develop a more severe form of ovarian hyperstimulation syndrome that can also cause rapid weight gain and shortness of breath.

- Miscarriage.

The rate of miscarriage for women who conceive using IVF with fresh embryos is similar to that of women who conceive naturally about 15% to 25% but the rate increases with maternal age.

- Egg-retrieval procedure complications.

Use of an aspirating needle to collect eggs could possibly cause bleeding, infection or damage to the bowel, bladder or a blood vessel. Risks are also associated with sedation and general anesthesia, if used.

- Ectopic pregnancy.

About 2% to 5% of women who use IVF will have an ectopic pregnancy when the fertilized egg implants outside the uterus, usually in a fallopian tube. The fertilized egg can't survive outside the uterus, and there's no way to continue the pregnancy.

-

- Birth defects.

The age of the mother is the primary risk factor in the development of birth defects, no matter how the child is conceived. More research is needed to determine whether babies conceived using IVF might be at increased risk of certain birth defects.

- Cancer.

Although some early studies suggested there may be a link between certain medications used to stimulate egg growth and the development of a specific type of ovarian tumor, more-recent studies do not support these findings. There does not appear to be a significantly increased risk of breast, endometrial, cervical or ovarian cancer after IVF.

- Stress.

Use of IVF can be financially, physically and emotionally draining. Support from counselors, family and friends can help you and your partner through the ups and downs of infertility treatment.

How You Prepare

The Centers for Disease Control and Prevention and the Society for Assisted Reproductive Technology provide information online about U.S. clinics' individual pregnancy and live birth rates.

When choosing an in vitro fertilization (IVF) clinic, keep in mind that a clinic's success rate depends on many factors, such as patients' ages and medical issues, as well as the clinic's treatment population and treatment approaches. Ask for detailed information about the costs associated with each step of the procedure.

Before beginning a cycle of IVF using your own eggs and sperm, you and your partner will likely need various screenings, including:

- Ovarian reserve testing.

To determine the quantity and quality of your eggs, your doctor might test the concentration of follicle-stimulating hormone (FSH), estradiol (estrogen) and anti-mullerian hormone in your blood during the first few days of your menstrual cycle. Test results, often used together with an ultrasound of your ovaries, can help predict how your ovaries will respond to fertility medication.

- Semen analysis.

If not done as part of your initial fertility evaluation, your doctor will conduct a semen analysis shortly before the start of an IVF treatment cycle.

- Infectious disease screening.

You and your partner will both be screened for infectious diseases, including HIV.

- Practice (mock) embryo transfer.

Your doctor might conduct a mock embryo transfer to determine the depth of your uterine cavity and the technique most likely to successfully place the embryos into your uterus.

- Uterine exam.

Your doctor will examine the inside lining of the uterus before you start IVF. This might involve a sonohysterography in which fluid is injected through the cervix into your uterus and an ultrasound to create images of your uterine cavity. Or it might include a hysteroscopy in which a thin, flexible, lighted telescope (hysteroscope) is inserted through your vagina and cervix into your uterus.

Before beginning a cycle of IVF, consider important questions

How many embryos will be transferred? The number of embryos transferred is typically based on age and number of eggs retrieved. Since the rate of implantation is lower for older women, more embryos are usually transferred except for women using donor eggs or genetically tested embryos.

Most doctors follow specific guidelines to prevent a higher order multiple pregnancy triplets or more and in some countries, legislation limits the number of embryos that can be transferred. Make sure you and your doctor agree on the number of embryos that will be transferred before the transfer procedure.

What will you do with any extra embryos? Extra embryos can be frozen and stored for future use for several years. Not all embryos will survive the freezing and thawing process, although most will.

Cryopreservation can make future cycles of IVF less expensive and less invasive. Or, you might be able to donate unused frozen embryos to another couple or a research facility. You might also choose to discard unused embryos.

How will you handle a multiple pregnancy? If more than one embryo is transferred to your uterus, IVF can result in a multiple pregnancy which poses health risks for you and your babies. In some cases, fetal reduction can be used to help a woman deliver fewer babies with lower health risks. Pursuing fetal reduction, however, is a major decision with ethical, emotional and psychological consequences.

Have you considered the potential complications associated with using donor eggs, sperm or embryos, or a gestational carrier? A trained counselor with expertise in donor issues can help you understand the concerns, such as the legal rights of the donor. You may also need an attorney to file court papers to help you become legal parents of an implanted embryo.

What you can expect

IVF involves several steps ovarian stimulation, egg retrieval, sperm retrieval, fertilization and embryo transfer. One cycle of IVF can take about two to three weeks, and more than one cycle may be required.

Ovulation Induction

If you're using your own eggs during IVF, at the start of a cycle you'll begin treatment with synthetic hormones to stimulate your ovaries to produce multiple eggs rather than the single egg that normally develops each month. Multiple eggs are needed because some eggs won't fertilize or develop normally after fertilization.

You may need several different medications, such as:

- Medications for ovarian stimulation.

To stimulate your ovaries, you might receive an injectable medication containing a follicle-stimulating hormone (FSH), a luteinizing hormone (LH) or a combination of both. These medications stimulate more than one egg to develop at a time.

- Medications for oocyte maturation.

When the follicles are ready for egg retrieval generally after eight to 14 days you will take human chorionic gonadotropin (HCG) or other medications to help the eggs mature.

- Medications to prevent premature ovulation.

These medications prevent your body from releasing the developing eggs too soon.

- Medications to prepare the lining of your uterus.

On the day of egg retrieval or at the time of embryo transfer, your doctor might recommend that you begin taking progesterone supplements to make the lining of your uterus more receptive to implantation.

Your doctor will work with you to determine which medications to use and when to use them.

Typically, you'll need one to two weeks of ovarian stimulation before your eggs are ready for retrieval. To determine when the eggs are ready for collection, your doctor will likely perform:

Vaginal ultrasound, an imaging exam of your ovaries to monitor the development of follicles fluid-filled ovarian sacs where eggs mature.

Blood tests, to measure your response to ovarian stimulation medications estrogen levels typically increase as follicles develop, and progesterone levels remain low until after ovulation

Sometimes IVF cycles need to be canceled before egg retrieval for one of these reasons:

- Inadequate number of follicles developing
- Premature ovulation
- Too many follicles developing, creating a risk of ovarian hyperstimulation syndrome

Other medical issues

If your cycle is canceled, your doctor might recommend changing medications or their doses to promote a better response during future IVF cycles. Or you may be advised that you need an egg donor.

Egg Retrieval

Egg retrieval can be done in your doctor's office or a clinic 34 to 36 hours after the final injection and before ovulation. During egg retrieval, you'll be sedated and given pain medication.

Transvaginal ultrasound aspiration is the usual retrieval method. An ultrasound probe is inserted into your vagina to identify follicles. Then a thin needle is inserted into an ultrasound guide to go through the vagina and into the follicles to retrieve the eggs.

If your ovaries aren't accessible through transvaginal ultrasound, an abdominal ultrasound may be used to guide the needle.

The eggs are removed from the follicles through a needle connected to a suction device. Multiple eggs can be removed in about 20 minutes.

After egg retrieval, you may experience cramping and feelings of fullness or pressure.

Mature eggs are placed in a nutritive liquid (culture medium) and incubated. Eggs that appear healthy and mature will be mixed with sperm to attempt to create embryos.

However, not all eggs may be successfully fertilized.

Sperm Retrieval

If you're using your partner's sperm, he'll provide a semen sample at your doctor's office or a clinic through masturbation the morning of egg retrieval. Other methods, such as testicular aspiration the use of a needle or surgical procedure to extract sperm directly from the testicle are sometimes required. Donor sperm also can be used. Sperm are separated from the semen fluid in the lab.

Fertilization

Fertilization can be attempted using two common methods:

- Conventional insemination. During conventional insemination, healthy sperm and mature eggs are mixed and incubated overnight.

- Intracytoplasmic sperm injection (ICSI). In ICSI, a single healthy sperm is injected directly into each mature egg. ICSI is often used when semen quality or number is a problem or if fertilization attempts during prior IVF cycles failed.

- In certain situations, your doctor may recommend other procedures before embryo transfer.

- Assisted hatching. About five to six days after fertilization, an embryo "hatches" from its surrounding membrane (zona pellucida), allowing it to implant into the lining of the uterus. If you're an older woman, or if you have had multiple failed IVF attempts, your doctor might recommend assisted hatching a technique in which a hole is made in the zona pellucida just before transfer to help the embryo hatch and implant. Assisted hatching is also useful for eggs or embryos that have been previously frozen as the process can harden the zona pellucida.

- Preimplantation genetic testing. Embryos are allowed to develop in the incubator until they reach a stage where a small sample can be removed and tested for specific genetic diseases or the correct number of chromosomes, typically after five to six days of development. Embryos that don't contain affected genes or chromosomes can be transferred to your uterus. While preimplantation genetic testing can reduce the likelihood that a parent will pass on a genetic problem, it can't eliminate the risk. Prenatal testing may still be recommended.

Embryo Transfer

Embryo transfer is done at your doctor's office or a clinic and usually takes place two to five days after egg retrieval.

You might be given a mild sedative. The procedure is usually painless, although you might experience mild cramping. The doctor will insert a long, thin, flexible tube called a catheter into your vagina, through your cervix and into your uterus.

A syringe containing one or more embryos suspended in a small amount of fluid is attached to the end of the catheter.

Using the syringe, the doctor places the embryo or embryos into your uterus. If successful, an embryo will implant in the lining of your uterus about six to 10 days after egg retrieval.

After the procedure

After the embryo transfer, you can resume normal daily activities. However, your ovaries may still be enlarged. Consider avoiding vigorous activity, which could cause discomfort.

Typical side effects include:

Passing a small amount of clear or bloody fluid shortly after the procedure due to the swabbing of the cervix before the embryo transfer.

- Breast tenderness due to high estrogen levels
- Mild bloating
- Mild cramping
- Constipation

If you develop moderate or svere pain after the embryo transfer, contact your doctor. He or she will evaluate you for complications such as infection, twisting of an ovary (ovarian torsion) and severe ovarian hyperstimulation syndrome.

About 12 days to two weeks after egg retrieval, your doctor will test a sample of your blood to detect whether you're pregnant.

If you're pregnant, your doctor will refer you to an obstetrician or other pregnancy specialist for prenatal care. If you're not pregnant, you'll stop taking progesterone and likely get your period within a week. If you don't get your period or you have unusual bleeding, contact your doctor. If you're interested in attempting another cycle of in vitro fertilization (IVF), your doctor might suggest steps you can take to improve your chances of getting pregnant through IVF. The chances of giving birth to a healthy baby after using IVF depend on various factors, including:

- Maternal age. The younger you are, the more likely you are to get pregnant and give birth to a healthy baby using your own eggs during IVF. Women age 41 and older are often counseled to consider using donor eggs during IVF to increase the chances of success.

- Embryo status. Transfer of embryos that are more developed is associated with higher pregnancy rates compared with less-developed embryos (day two or three). However, not all embryos survive the development process. Talk with your doctor or other care provider about your specific situation.

- Reproductive history. Women who've previously given birth are more likely to be able to get pregnant using IVF than are women who've never given birth. Success rates are lower for women who've previously used IVF multiple times but didn't get pregnant.

- Cause of infertility. Having a normal supply of eggs increases your chances of being able to get pregnant using IVF. Women who have severe endometriosis are less likely to be able to get pregnant using IVF than are women who have unexplained infertility.

- Lifestyle factors. Women who smoke typically have fewer eggs retrieved during IVF and may miscarry more often. Smoking can lower a woman's chance of success using IVF by 50%. Obesity can decrease your chances of getting pregnant and having a baby. Use of alcohol, recreational drugs, excessive caffeine and certain medications also can be harmful.

Talk with your doctor about any factors that apply to you and how they may affect your chances of a successful pregnancy.

IVF Diet: Foods To Eat And Foods To Avoid During Treatment

Before starting with the IVF Diet you need to know this; there is no proven result of what you eat helps you infertility treatment however what you eat has a relation with your health and that affects the healthy egg or sperm. And to get a healthy pregnancy, it is very important that sperm and eggs should be healthy which does not has a direct connection with your food intake but yes it does has a connection with the type of food we consume.

Once you have decided to go for the IVF treatment, start monitoring your diet. It is seen that obesity or too low body weight affects fertility adversely and reduces the success rate of IVF. So, starting with an excellent diet will be a great option to fight these issues. Paying attention to your diet and essential nutrients will help your body to carry pregnancy easily. The IVF process is emotionally and physically demanding, so a good diet is also a way to boost up your mood and be relax by the medium of food. Enjoy your food at fullest and along with getting its benefits, you will be stress- free.

Everyone has a different body type so no diet is perfect for the same group of people. But getting a diet plan is not a bad idea. The diet plan will include food based on the researches through which we know which food is good and what to avoid during IVF treatment.

Healthy eating is a means of getting the desired amount of macros for your body every day. So list down the things by making two lists: what to eat and what not to eat and put it somewhere in front of you as a reminder. Along with having healthy and balanced diet meals, it is also important to track your calories. So you can use a mobile application to track your calories. Tracking your nutrition will definitely allow you to see what is working and what is not working for you and meanwhile, you can make changes to your diet, and bring out the best diet for IVF success for yourself.

Food to eat during IVF treatment.

By understanding your food, you will have a better chance of Pregnancy IVF success as food has an indirect relation with the process and the right choice of food will help your body to respond in a better way. Although your doctor will not provide you the list of the food you should take, it is necessary to understand the process.

There are certain nutrients which are essential for the IVF treatment to be a success.

Food rich in zinc: If your hormones that are responsible for the regulation of the reproduction process in the body are at an appropriate level, it will affect the entire process in an effective way. Any kind of hormonal imbalance will cause an unpredictable functioning of ovaries or eggs. Zinc helps in balancing the hormone level. Therefore, to meet the daily requirement of zinc which is 15 mg will work to benefit you. You can also rely on zinc supplements but natural ways of consuming nutrients are considered better. Include grains, nuts, dairy products, meat items and potatoes which are rich in zinc.

Folic acid in food: A pregnancy superhero! Yes, you heard it right, folic acid is considered a superhero for your pregnancy. Folic acid along with certain parental vitamins helps in the healthy development of a child's brain and spinal cord. Generally, birth defects occur in the first 3-4 weeks of pregnancy due to lack of certain nutrients in the body required for the development of a child. So, you can store the amount of folate in your body to ensure proper brain and spinal cord development.

How much folic acid you should consume on a daily basis while you are planning a baby

- When you plan and try to conceive: 400 mcg

- In the first 3 months of pregnancy: 400 mcg

- In the 4th-9th month of pregnancy: 600 mcg

- Iron-rich food:

Boost up the iron storage of your body, as having an iron deficiency or anemia can cause your baby to born too early or too small. Every month during menstruation, women lose iron and due to lack of a healthy diet, many of them suffer from iron deficiency. Iron in the body is related to ovulation and good health of eggs; Deficiency of iron leads to poor egg health.

Ensure adding iron-rich food in your diet like Pumpkin seeds, oysters and spinach. For vegetarian people, you can add iron supplements in your diet but after consulting your doctor.

- Healthy fats

If fats are consumed in moderation, it is actually beneficial for your body. But trans-saturated fats which are present in junk foods should be avoided at any cost. Consuming fats from walnuts, olive oil, corn, chia seeds, and flaxseed oil are healthy fatty acid and are unsaturated fats which are recommended because these help in the formation of healthy eggs in your body. These fats will work as energy storage in your body which you might need in the journey of IVF treatment and after a successful pregnancy.

- Protein-rich food

Appropriate presence of protein in your body affects the development of eggs in the ovaries. Protein is highly recommended in the process of getting pregnant as it helps in the development of the body and provides instant energy to the body. It is necessary to include 60 gram of protein in your diet on a daily basis. Eggs, meat, and dairy products are a great source of protein.

- Hydration for the body

With today's lifestyle, drinking enough water required for your body has become a task. We forget to drink water and our body has to suffer because of that. The optimal level of water in our body is connected to maintain a good balance between different elements of the body. Water supports circulation also. So, make it a ritual to drink the required amount of water every day; neither less nor more, just the perfect amount needed by your body.

Now after getting an overview of food that increases fertility, let us have a glance of food items that you need to include and avoid during this process. Keep your health at its best to increase the success rate of the IVF.

Food to eat during the treatment

- Green Leafy Vegetables: Green leafy vegetable is on the top because these are fertility boosting food. As these are rich in antioxidants, folic acid, and iron, they should a be part of your daily food intake.

- Cabbage: Loaded with essential vitamin and minerals, the Di-indole methane present in cabbage helps in regulating estrogen metabolism.

- Broccoli: As broccoli is rich in Vitamin C, it assists in maturing the eggs. Along with that rich iron content, anti-oxidants, and folic acid helps in the proper development of your body and fetus.

- Potatoes: Potatoes helps to increase the cell division in the body. Regular consumption of potatoes provides essential vitamins like B and E to your body.

- Banana: Loaded with vitamin B6, this superfood helps in regulating menstruation cycles. You can consider this fruit as a healthy snack option because it provides you with versatile options.

- •Pineapple: Pineapple contains a good amount of manganese in it. Manganese is known as a reproductive mineral and so it helps in boosting the reproductive hormones.

- Salmon: Rich content of Omega-3 fatty acids makes this food an essential intake because it can help in Oestrogen balance and also increase blood flow. It should be properly cooked

- Complex Carbs: Complex carbs are great for regulating blood sugar level. It will also help you in maintaining a healthy weight.

- Colorful Fruits and Vegetables: Colors in fruits and vegetable has its own significance. They are loaded with essential nutrients.

Food to avoid during the treatment

Eggs in raw form: Raw form of eggs are used in many food products like mayonnaise, biscuit cream, and salad dressing. But there is a virus named salmonella virus which is present in raw eggs which can cause food poisoning. Hence, it is recommended to avoid consuming eggs in raw form. Cook it well before you eat.

• Artificial sweeteners: Avoid consuming food that comes with artificial sweeteners. It is bad for your health in the normal state also. Saccharin based sweeteners reduce the success rate of IVF. Instead, you can use sucralose-based sweeteners or any natural sweetening syrup.

• Refined sugars: Food containing refined sugar in it makes you feel happy for some time but pressurize liver to produce more insulin quickly to balance the sugar level. These pressure over the organs of the body begins to affect the fertility process.

• Seafood: Seafood is a good source of protein and essential fatty acid but consuming raw or half-cooked seafood causes infection. Also, seafood is rich in mercury content which causes issues with the development of the fetus and result in birth defects.

•   Alcohol: Alcohol is the major cause of erratic ovulation in women. It does not only affect the health of eggs but is also responsible for the fetus impairment.

• Caffeine: Limit the amount of coffee and tea when you are going under the process of IVF.

• Cheese: Not all cheese but specific types of cheese should be avoided. Few varieties of cheese contain bacteria known for causing infection.

Supplements To Increase Fertility

A well-balanced diet will provide you with nearly everything you need for your pregnancy. However, the National Institute of Health and Care Excellence (NICE) recommend that women supplement their diet with two extra vitamins around the time of conception.

Folate

(the natural form of folic acid) is a B-vitamin. It occurs naturally in dark green leafy vegetables, fruits, dairy products and seafood. Low folate status is common in the UK, and if it occurs during pregnancy it can have a negative impact on babies. They may be born small for their age or have birth defects. The most common defects related to low folate are neural tube defects such as spina bifida.

All women in the UK are advised to take 400ug of folic acid 8 weeks prior to conception. They should then continue taking it up to 12 weeks of pregnancy. This is to ensure there is a good folic acid supply at conception and until the neural tube closes.

Vitamin D

Similarly to folate, vitamin D deficiency is common in the UK. It plays an important role in our bodies, helping with the absorption of dietary calcium and phosphate from our intestines. These three nutrients are needed to help maintain healthy bones, teeth and muscles. They are also key to the development of your baby during pregnancy.

NICE recommend that all women take a daily supplement of 10ug from conception all the way through their pregnancy. It is also recommended to continue supplementation throughout breastfeeding as well, to ensure there is an adequate supply in breastmilk.

Your 7-Day Pregnancy Meal Plan

- **Monday**

Breakfast

- Low-Gi muesli
- Natural yoghurt
- Few slices of your favourite fruit

Lunch

Chicken salad with avocado, leafy green veggies and cheese with a balsamic and olive oil dressing.

Dinner

A non-fatty steak, with a fresh mushroom sauce and spinach.

Snack option

Boiled egg

- **Tuesday**

Breakfast

Boiled or poached egg on wholewheat bread with slices of avocado.

Lunch

Vegetable wrap including red, green and yellow peppers, grated carrots, lettuce, tomato and some humus.

Dinner

Chicken fillets stuffed with feta cheese and a side of vegetables.

Snack option

Cracker breads with cottage cheese.

- **Wednesday**

Breakfast

Breakfast wrap filled with scrambled eggs, tomato and feta or mozzarella cheese - your choice.

Lunch

Chicken mayonnaise toasted sandwich on health bread.

Dinner

Pizza with whole-wheat crust, topped with fresh tomatoes and veggies of your choice.

Snack option

Home-made air popcorn.

- **Thursday**

Breakfast

Breakfast oats wiht honey and a fruit on the side.

Lunch

Vegetable soup for those overcast days. Throw as many veggies in the pot as possible.

Dinner

Either a meat or vegetable stew with brown rice.

Snack option

Oat bars.

- **Friday**

Breakfast

Ready-made whole-wheat waffles, with fruit and honey on top.

Lunch

Couscous salad with cucumber, tomato and other veggies you may want to add in.

Dinner

Vegetable sushi (no raw fish in it whatsoever) for a night out meal.

Snack option

Carrots and cucumber with hummus dip.

- **Saturday**

Breakfast

Bran cereal with two-percent fat milk with sliced banana on top.

Lunch

Baked potato with cottage cheese and chives on top.

Dinner

Vegetable, meat or chicken tacos with an assortment of veggies and sprinkled with cheese.

Snack option

Smoothies with left over yoghurt and fruit.

- **Sunday**

Breakfast

Whole-wheat toast with peanut butter and a fresh fruit on the side.

Lunch

Pasta salad with added mushrooms, peppers and mozarella.

Dinner

Hake fillets, with a lemon butter sauce, a side of baked potato and a green salad.

Snack option

Fruit.

IVF Meal Recipes

Simple Baked Salmon

A quick and easy dish that requires very little effort. It works best with fresh salmon purchased the same day you plan to eat it.

Place the salmon filets on a large piece of aluminum foil in a glass baking dish. Slice the butter into pats and put then evenly spaced on top of the salmon. Wrap the foil over the top of the fish and crimp along the sides to seal somewhat tightly.

Bake in a 350 degree oven for 15-30 minutes depending on the thickness of the filets. You want them to be cooked until they start to flake and become opaque inside, but don't dry them out.

Serve with tartar sauce and your choice of salad.

Awesome Almond Buckwheat Pancakes
Ingredients / Directions

- 1/3 c buckwheat flour
- 1/3 c whole wheat (or whole spelt) flour
- 3/4 tsp baking powder
- 1/4 tsp salt
- 2 tsp sugar (optional)

Combine separately:
- 1/3 c yogurt
- 1/2 c milk (or milk substitute)
- 1 egg

- 1 Tbsp melted butter

Direction

- Mix wet and dry ingredients until just incorporated - batter can be a bit lumpy.

- Heat a frying pan over medium heat with about a teaspoon of butter. Pour in 1/4 of the batter and generously sprinkle with slivered almonds. When bubbles start to appear in your pancake, flip it and cook untill slightly browned on bottom. Repeat with the rest of the batter adding a bit more butter to the pan each time.

- Serve warm with maple syrup.

Servings: 4

Bircher Muesli

Ingredients

- (2 servings)   Printable Version

- 1/2 cup oatmeal

- 1/4 cup Apple Juice

- 1/4 cup natural plain or vanilla yogurt

- Pinch of cinnamon

- 1 medium apple (preferably Granny Smith)

- 1 Tablespoon crushed almonds

- 1 Tablespoon dried cranberries

- 1 medium banana

- 1 handful blueberries

Direction

- Mix oatmeal, juice, cinnamon and yogurt together in a large bowl. Cover and refrigerate overnight.

- In the morning, grate the apple and slice the banana into the oatmeal. Mix in the blueberries, almonds and cranberries.

- Enjoy!

Mushroom And Herb Omelet

Ingredients

- (2 servings)   Printable Version

- 4 large eggs

- 1 and 1/2 cups fresh mushrooms - sliced

- 1 tablespoon fresh parsley - chopped

- 1 teaspoon fresh oregano

- Basil or thyme - finely chopped

- 2 teaspoons butter

- Salt and pepper to taste

Direction

- In small bowl, wisk together eggs and spices. Set aside.

- In a medium skillet at just above medium heat, saute the mushrooms in half the butter (1 teaspoon) until tender; set aside.

- In same skillet, melt half of the remaining butter (1/2 teaspoon). Pour half of the egg mixture into skillet. Cook, lifting edge to allow uncooked portion to flow underneath. When almost set, spoon half of the mushrooms over half of the omelet. Fold other half over the mushrooms; slide onto a serving plate.

California Plum and Quinoa Salad
Ingredients

- 1 1/4 cups quinoa
- 2 1/2 cups water
- 2 fresh California plums, pitted and diced
- 1/2 cup chopped, toasted walnuts
- 1/4 cup chopped red bell pepper
- 1/4 cup chopped yellow bell pepper
- 1/4 cup sliced green onions
- 3 tablespoons flax oil
- 3 tablespoons extra-virgin olive oil
- 1/4 cup white wine vinegar
- 1 1/2 tablespoons honey
- 1/4 teaspoon salt

Directions

Rinse quinoa and drain well. Add to boiling water; reduce heat and simmer, covered, for 12 minutes. Remove from heat and let stand for 5 minutes. Fluff with a fork and let chill for about 30 minutes. Stir together quinoa, plums, walnuts, peppers and onions in a medium bowl. Whisk together remaining ingredients in a small bowl and pour over salad; toss well to coat all ingredients with dressing. Cover and chill for 1 hour.

Garbanzo Bean and Quinoa Salad

Ingredients

- 1 cup quinoa

- 2 cups water

- 1 (15 ounce) can garbanzo beans, drained

- 1/2 cup dried cranberries

- 1/2 cup golden raisins

- 1/3 cup sliced almonds

- 1/4 cup mint leaves, chopped

- 3/4 teaspoon ground coriander

- 1/4 teaspoon ground cumin

- 1 tablespoon extra-virgin olive oil

- Salt and pepper to taste

Directions

Bring the quinoa and water to a boil in a saucepan over high heat. Reduce heat to medium-low, cover, and simmer until the quinoa is tender, and the water has been absorbed, 15 to 20 minutes. Scrape the quinoa into a large bowl, and refrigerate until cold.

Stir the garbanzo beans, cranberries, raisins, almonds, mint, coriander, cumin, and olive oil into the quinoa. Season to taste with salt and pepper.

Curried Quinoa Salad with Mango
Ingredients
- 1 1/2 cups chicken stock
- 3/4 cup quinoa
- 1 1/2 teaspoons curry powder
- 1/4 teaspoon garlic powder
- 1/2 teaspoon salt
- 1/4 teaspoon black pepper
- 1 mango - peeled, seeded and diced
- 3 green onions, chopped

Directions
Bring chicken stock, quinoa, curry powder, garlic powder, salt, and pepper to a boil in a saucepan over high heat. Reduce heat to medium-low, cover, and simmer

until the quinoa is tender, 15 to 20 minutes. Once done, scrape the quinoa into a shallow dish and allow to cool to room temperature. Stir in the mango and green onions.

Serve either at room temperature or cold.

Quinoa with Veggies

Ingredients
- 1 cup quinoa
- 3 cups water
- 1 pinch salt
- 3 tablespoons olive oil
- 3 cloves garlic, minced
- 1 red bell pepper, chopped
- 1/2 cup corn kernels
- 1/2 teaspoon cumin
- 1 teaspoon dried oregano
- Salt and pepper to taste
- 2 green onions, chopped

Directions

- Bring the quinoa, water, and 1 pinch of salt to a boil in a saucepan. Reduce heat to medium-low, cover, and simmer until the quinoa is tender, about 20 minutes. Once done, drain a mesh strainer, and set aside.

- Meanwhile, heat the olive oil in a saucepan over medium heat. Stir in the garlic, and cook until the garlic softens and the aroma mellows, about 2 minutes. Add the red pepper, and corn; continue cooking until the pepper softens, about 5 minutes. Season with cumin, oregano, salt, and pepper, and cook for 1 minute more, then stir in the cooked quinoa and green onions. Serve hot or cold.

Chile Garlic BBQ Salmon

Ingredients

- 3 pounds whole salmon, cleaned

- 1/4 cup soy sauce

- 1 tablespoon chile sauce

- 1 tablespoon chopped fresh ginger root

- 1 clove garlic, chopped
- 1 lime, juiced
- 1 lime, zested
- 1 tablespoon brown sugar
- 3 green onions, chopped

Directions
- Trim the tail and fins off of the salmon. Make several shallow cuts across the salmon's skin. Place salmon on 3 large, slightly overlapping sheets of aluminum foil.
- In a bowl, stir together soy sauce, chile sauce, ginger, and garlic. Mix in lime juice, lime zest, and brown sugar. Spoon sauce over the salmon.
- Fold the foil over the salmon, and crimp the edges to seal.
- If using hot coals, move them to one side of the grill. Place the fish on the side of the grill that does not have coals directly underneath it, and close the lid. If using a gas grill, place the fish on one side, and turn off the flames directly underneath it; close the lid. Cook for 25 to 30

minutes. Remove to a serving platter, and pour any juices that may have collected in the foil over the top of the fish. Sprinkle with green onions.

Aromatic salmon cooked in coconut milk
Preparation time less than 30 mins

Cooking time 30 mins to 1 hour

Serves 4

Ingredients
- 4 thick salmon steaks
- 2.5cm/1in piece root ginger, peeled and cut into small, very thin slices
- 2 large cloves garlic, peeled and cut into small, very thin slices
- 350g/12oz tomatoes, peeled and halved
- 1 fresh red chilli, de-seeded and sliced as finely as possible
- 1 small yellow pepper, de-seeded and thinly sliced
- 4-6 cardamom pods, roughly crushed

- 400ml/14fl oz tinned coconut milk

- Sea salt

- 2 limes, juice only

- Handful of fresh mint leaves, chopped

Method

- Put the fish steaks in a fairly shallow ovenproof dish with a lid, into which they fit quite closely.

- Scatter the ginger, garlic, tomato, chilli and yellow pepper over and around the fish and the cardamom pods in between.

- Empty the coconut milk into a separate bowl, add a good sprinkling of sea salt and gradually stir in the lime juice. Pour the mixture gently over and around the fish and cover the dish.

- Preheat the oven to 150C/300F/Gas 2. Put the dish on the centre shelf and cook for 40-50 minutes, until the fish is lightly done. To discover this insert a small, sharp knife into the centre of one of the steaks if the flesh is slightly darker pink in the centre it will be perfectly cooked. Remove from the oven.

- Before serving scatter the mint leaves on top.

Ham and Potato Soup Recipe

Ingredients:

- 3 large potatoes, peeled and diced

- 1-2 cups cooked ham, cut into small pieces

- 1/2 cup half & half

- 3-4 cups chicken stock

- 3-4 chicken bouillon cubes

- 1 onion, diced

- 1/2 cup butter

- 1/2 cup flour

- Salt and pepper to taste

Direction

- Put diced potatoes in a cooking pot and add approximately 3 cups of water. You will save this cooking water and add it to the soup pot later, so use just enough to cover the potatoes. Add 1-2 bouillon cubes for flavor. Bring water to a boil and cook long enough for the potatoes to be tender without being mushy, approximately 15 minutes.

- Transfer cooked potatoes and water to a larger soup pot or crock pot. Add ham and half & half to the crock pot, stir and begin heating all. While potatoes are boiling, chop the onion.

- Melt butter in a heavy bottomed skillet. Saute the onion for a few minutes until the onion is just beginning to turn golden.

- Add the flour to the onion and butter mixture and cook for 5 minutes over medium heat. This will be a very thick paste. Stir occasionally to prevent burning.

- Gradually stir in approximately 3 cups of liquid. This liquid can be chicken or turkey stock if on-hand, else use water with chicken bouillon. Stir frequently and cook over medium heat for approximately 10 minutes. The sauce should be thick and bubbly.

- Transfer the thick sauce into the crock pot with the other ingredients, stir and adjust seasoning. Ham is usually pretty salty, so be cautious about adding extra salt.

- Soup can be served as soon as it is hot or allowed to simmer on low in the crock pot until later.

Guacamole Recipe

Ingredients:

- 2 ripe avocados

- 1/2 ripe tomato, diced

- 1/2 white onion, diced

- 2-3 cloves finely chopped garlic

- finely diced fresh jalapeno pepper

- 2 tbsp chopped cilantro leaves

- 1/2 a fresh lime

- salt to taste

Direction

- High-quality avocados are the key to the recipe. Make sure to plan ahead to give them time to ripen. Cut avocados in half lengthwise with a chef's knife. Style points are given for sticking the knife into the pit like an axe blade and then twisting to remove. Scoop out with a big spoon and place in a large bowl. Using a knife and spoon, chop the avocado into 5mm pieces.

- Chop garlic, dice tomato, cut up onion, jalapeno pepper and cilantro and add all to the avocados.
- Squeeze lime juice on top, add salt to taste and mix.
- Serve in a molcajete with fresh tortilla chips and a frozen margarita.

Conclusion

Infertile women with greater adherence to Mediterranean diet pattern were likely to obtain more embryos available in IVF cycle.

While there is a well-characterized association between high intake of folic acid, polyunsaturated fats, and plant-based foods on fertility outcomes, further research is required to more clearly understand the roles of other foods. Future research should also consider the need for randomized controlled trials and studies examining the combined effects of diets of both male and female partners on fertility. Despite recent progress in the amount of literature on the relationship between fertility and diet. Thus, there is a need for more standardized integration of nutrition counseling into treatment delivery for infertility. Incorporating specific guidelines for individuals of reproductive age when developing federal nutritional guidelines may also impact the reach of this information. Furthermore, there is an urgent need to develop targeted messaging and interventions among individuals with extreme BMI categories, racial/ethnic minorities, and

low-income and low-education groups in order to improve existing disparities in both fertility and overall health outcomes in the U.S.

Given the positive effect of a healthy diet on fertility outcomes, and the implications for public health and clinical practice noted above, several recommendations can be noted. First, clinicians should provide counseling to improve dietary behaviors among patients accessing ART services, regardless of BMI while prioritizing those with unfavorable BMI. Specifically, a diet consistent with the U.S. Dietary Guidelines for Americans and adequate levels of folic acid intake for women could be recommended. Moreover, patients with a BMI consistent with underweight, overweight, or obesity status should be referred to nutritional and weight-loss counseling to help improve the likelihood of positive fertility outcomes. In order for health care providers to have the best and most current information on the effects of specific dietary components on fertility, there should be clear and effective communication between researchers and clinicians.

A second recommendation is to improve the delivery of nutritional programs and interventions aimed at the general reproductive-aged population, as well as targeted at-risk groups. For example, considering accessibility of an intervention has been cited as an important factor contributing to young adults' willingness to participate in a weight loss program. Thus, leveraging the ubiquity of mobile technology, such as text messaging or a Smartphone application, to deliver a healthy eating or weight loss intervention has been shown to be an effective strategy to engage this sector of the population. Given the sociodemographic and racial/ethnic disparities in infertility, efforts to improve the diets of reproductive-aged adults should target low socioeconomic or education groups and racial/ethnic minority populations. Interventions should consider the unique barriers these groups face related to optimal nutrition, including structural barriers such as access to healthy foods in terms of geographic accessibility as well as price.

Approaches that considers the structural barriers to a healthy diet among this target population may involve limiting the extent to which the U.S. government-assisted food benefit program Supplemental Nutrition Assistance Program can be used to purchase foods that contribute to infertility, such as sugary beverages, or incentivizing the purchase of foods consistent with a healthy diet pattern for reproductive-aged adults through a program similar to the Healthy Incentive Program.

In order to lend further support to fertility-promoting diets for the population, a third recommendation is to include evidence-based messaging in population-wide nutritional guidelines such as the U.S. Dietary Guidelines for Americans. The public health implications of nutrition and fertility in the U.S. are multifaceted. Future research and collaboration across stakeholders in research institutions, clinical practice, and the community will help drive and implement more evidence-based recommendations and interventions.

www.ingramcontent.com/pod-product-compliance
Lightning Source LLC
Chambersburg PA
CBHW050809160726
48004CB00002B/763